Mariana Aquino Holanda Pinto
Moacyr Oliveira Neto
Ianna Lacerda Sampaio Braga

Polypharmacy among the elderly in two healthcare institutions

Mariana Aquino Holanda Pinto
Moacyr Oliveira Neto
Ianna Lacerda Sampaio Braga

Polypharmacy among the elderly in two healthcare institutions

A descriptive and comparative study in Fortaleza, Ceará

ScienciaScripts

Imprint

Cover image: www.ingimage.com

This book is a translation from the original published under ISBN 978-3-330-99833-9.

Publisher:
Sciencia Scripts
is a trademark of
Dodo Books Indian Ocean Ltd. and OmniScriptum S.R.L publishing group

120 High Road, East Finchley, London, N2 9ED, United Kingdom
Str. Armeneasca 28/1, office 1, Chisinau MD-2012, Republic of Moldova, Europe
Managing Directors: Ieva Konstantinova, Victoria Ursu
info@omniscriptum.com

Printed at: see last page
ISBN: 978-620-8-64465-9

SUMMARY

Mariana Aquino Holanda Pinto[1], Moacyr Oliveira Neto[2], Ianna Lacerda Sampaio Braga[3]

1 Medical student at the University of Fortaleza (Unifor), PROBIC-FEQ scholarship holder.

2 Graduating in medicine from the Christus University Centre (Unichristus).

3 Geriatrician qualified by the National Council for Medical Residency (CNRM) and the Brazilian Society of Geriatrics and Gerontology (SBGG). Professor of Medicine at Unifor. Doctor at the Dr César Cals General Hospital, Ceará State Health Department (SESA/CE). PhD student at RENORBIO.

SUMMARY

Introduction: The elderly represent the fastest growing age group in Brazil, making their demand for health resources more intense, both in terms of the utilisation of services the use of medication.

Due to the prevalence of chronic degenerative diseases and various other comorbidities, polypharmacy has become a frequent practice and a major problem in the health care of the elderly.

The aim of this study was to describe and compare the prevalence of polypharmacy and the use of inappropriate medication in institutionalised elderly people and elderly people receiving outpatient care, and to correlate them with the clinical-epidemiological and socioeconomic profiles of each patient. Materials and methods: A descriptive cross-sectional study carried out by analysing medical records and applying a questionnaire to elderly patients treated at the Núcleo de Atenção Médica Integrada (Nami) and the Lar Torres de Melo (LTM) long-stay institution in Fortaleza, Ceará. Results: A sample of 150 elderly people was obtained: 100 institutionalised and 50 treated on an outpatient basis. The majority were female (54%), aged between 60 and 74 years (63.33%) with a minimum age of 60 and a maximum of 91.

Polypharmacy was observed in 60 per cent of the total sample. The elderly in the long-stay institution practised more polypharmacy than those in the community (63% versus 54%). The average number of medicines used per patient was 5.2.

The factors that showed a statistically significant relationship with polypharmacy were female gender, not having a partner, lower monthly income, lower schooling, not working and self-medication. 22% of the sample used medicines that were unsuitable for the elderly, and this practice was more common among the elderly in the community (28% versus 19%). 11 different inappropriate medicines were used by the sample, most of them related to the central nervous system.

We also found that 53.33% of the population used teas, herbs and home-made medicines. Conclusion: Polypharmacy was more common among institutionalised elderly people, but the use of inappropriate medication was more prevalent among community-dwelling elderly people. This study contributes to expanding knowledge about the profile of medication use in the population studied, providing data that should help in the management and prevention of polypharmacy and its consequences for the health of the elderly.

Keywords: Elderly health. Use of medication. Long-stay institution for the elderly. Potentially inappropriate medication.

CHAPTER 1

INTRODUCTION

Population ageing is a worldwide phenomenon that represents an increase in the elderly population in relation to other age groups. This growth is one of the major public health challenges in Brazil (DAL PIZZOL et al., 2012).

Along with this change in age, epidemiological changes are also being seen, with the main causes of death being parasitic and infectious diseases, replaced by chronic non-communicable diseases, which generally require ongoing human and drug assistance (CARVALHO et al., 2012).

The simultaneous involvement of several chronic diseases in an individual predisposes them to the association of several medicines, increasing the incidence of a condition called polypharmacy, defined by the use of five or more medicines simultaneously for at least a week or more medicines than are clinically necessary (DIEDERICHS; BERGER; BARTELS, 2011; FLORES; MENGUE, 2005; TAYLOR et al., 2010).

Regardless of age, the high consumption of medicines always involves risks for the consumer (ALMEIDA et al.,

1999). For frail elderly people, these risks become even greater, as their bodies undergo pharmacokinetic and pharmacodynamic changes typical of ageing, which, added to the lack of knowledge about the effect of drugs on the elderly, make this section of the population even more vulnerable to adverse effects and drug interactions (MARIN et al., 2010).

Polypharmacy is therefore one of the main factors correlated with iatrogenesis, with a strong and relevant relationship with the likelihood of adverse effects and the use of medicines contraindicated for the elderly (PASSARELLI; JACOB-FILHO; FIGUERAS, 2005).

The Beers - Fick criteria are a list of potentially inappropriate drugs for adults aged 65 and over, with the aim of detecting and avoiding potential risks of drug iatrogenesis (BEERS, 1997; BEERS et al., 1991; FICK et al., 2003).

Institutionalised elderly people are those most at risk of polypharmacy, since they have more limiting illnesses, greater frailty and lower functionality than those in the community, and main factors positively related to polypharmacy are the presence of dementia, the number of diagnoses and length of institutionalisation. In community-dwelling elderly people, gender and age are the factors most related to the use of many medicines (LUCCHETTI et al., 2010).

Finally, this study aims to characterise two groups: institutionalised elderly people and elderly people with outpatient medical care in Fortaleza, Ceará, in terms of their use of medication, verifying the existence of polypharmacy among them, seeking to correlate this prevalence with the clinical and epidemiological profiles of each group and to identify their risk factors.

CHAPTER 2

MATERIALS AND METHODS

This is an epidemiological, cross-sectional and observational study carried out by applying a questionnaire and analysing the medical records of 50 elderly patients assisted at the Núcleo de Atenção Médica Integrada (Nami) (Image 1), an outpatient medical care centre at the University of Fortaleza, and 100 elderly patients living in a non-governmental long-stay institution in Fortaleza, Lar Torres de Melo (LTM) (Image 2), selected by convenience sampling.

Data was collected between October 2014 and December 2015. The study included elderly people aged 60 or over who were able to answer the questionnaire and who consented to take part.

Of the total number of candidates in the initial sample, two elderly people did not consent to take part in the study, 12 were not cognitively able to answer the questionnaire and four were unable to provide information about the medications they were taking, so they were excluded from the study.

The questionnaires were administered in a targeted interview by two previously trained interviewers, and a total of 150 forms were answered in full.

The data was collected in a database in the EPIDATA 3.1 programme with identification information such as gender, age group, marital status and schooling, clinical characteristics of each patient such as diagnosed illnesses, prescription and quantity of medication and each patient's self-reported perception of health.

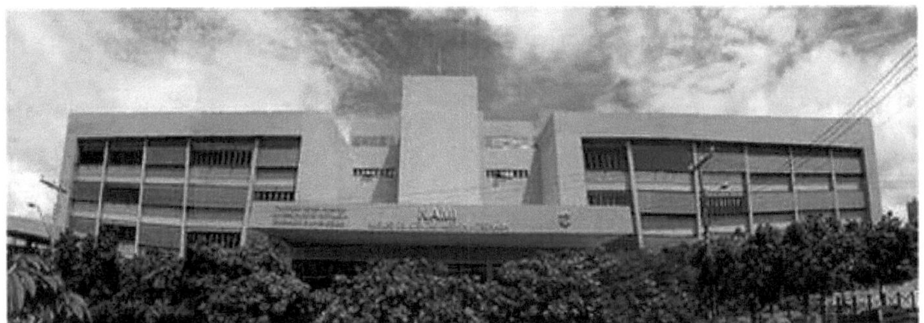

Image 1 - Integrated Medical Care Centre (Nami), a secondary health care institution in Fortaleza, CE.

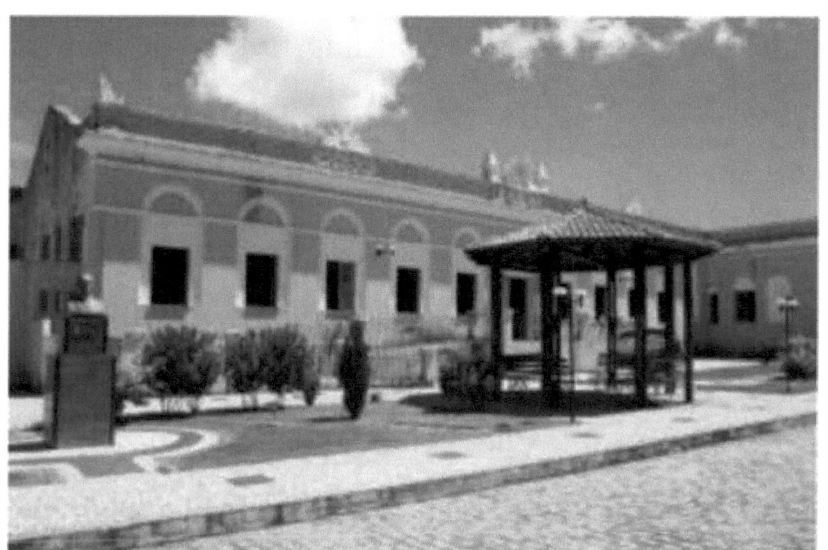

Image 2: Lar Torres de Melo (LTM), a long-stay institution for the elderly and primary health care centre in Fortaleza, CE.

Polypharmacy was considered to be the simultaneous use of five or more medicines (MEDEIROS SOUZA et al., 2007; SILVIA REGINA, 2010) for a minimum period of one week.

Based on this analysis, each elderly person was characterised in terms of their use of medication and the practice of polypharmacy. The main chronic diseases reported were grouped according to the International Classification of Diseases (ICD-10) (WHO, 1995).

The medicines most used by patients with

polypharmacy were classified according to the Anatomical Therapeutic Chemical Code (ATCC), adopted by the World Health Organisation (WHO) (WHO, 2006).

The Beers - Fick Criterion was used to classify the drug as inappropriate for the elderly according to the active ingredient and the data was analysed using SPSS 22 and EpiInfo 7.0.

The research was authorised by the coordinator of the LTM and the director of the Nami by signing the Letters of Consent and the Terms of Trust and approved by the Unifor Research Ethics Committee under number 953.397, in compliance with the Norms and Regulatory Guidelines for Research Involving Human Beings - Res.466/12 CNS/MS.

CHAPTER 3

RESULTS

Of the 150 elderly people interviewed, the majority were female (54%), aged between 60 and 74 (63.3%) with a minimum age of 60 and a maximum of 91, had studied for 5 to 8 years (45.33%), did not have a partner (85.3%), received an income of up to 1 minimum wage (74.3%) and did not work (87.3%) (Table 1).

The majority rated their health as very good or good (46.7%) or fair (36%), 32.7% of the elderly reported having fallen and 14% having been hospitalised at least once in the last 12 months prior to the survey and, with regard to comorbidities, 75.3% reported having between 1 and 3 chronic diseases.

148 elderly people were taking medication and the total number of medications was 784. No medication was used up to a maximum of 14 per patient, giving an average of 5.2 medications per patient.

With regard to the number of medicines, the majority of elderly people (57.33%) used between 1 and 5 medicines, , and polypharmacy was observed in 60% of cases.

Table 1 - Socio-demographic data of the elderly participating in the study (n=150) in Fortaleza, CE 2016.

	Institutionalised		Not institutionalised		Total		P-value
	N	%	N	%	N	%	
Sex							p=0.0001*
Female	43	43%	38	76%	81	54%	
Male	57	57%	12	24%	69	46%	
Age group							
60 a 74	58	58%	37	74%	95	63,3%	p=0.0213
75 or more	42	42%	13	26%	55	36,7 %	
Education							
Did not study	28	28%	6	12%	34	22,7 %	
up to 4 years	19	19%	6	12%	25	16,7 %	p=0.02
5 to 8 years	37	37%	31	72%	68	45,3 %	
more than 8 years	16	16%	7	14%	23	15,3 %	
Marital status							
No mate	93	93%	35	70%	128	85,3%	p=0.002*
With a mate	7	7%	15	30%	22	14,7%	
Income							
Up to 1 salary	81	85,26%	23	51,11 %	104	74,3%	p<0.0001*
> of 1 salary	14	14,74%	22	48,89 %	36	25,71%	
Working conditions							
Inactive	92	92%	39	78%	131	87.3%	p=0.015
Active	8	8%	11	22%	19	12,67%	

Source: PINTO; OLIVEIRA NETO; BRAGA, 2017.

Table 2 - Health status indicators of the elderly participating in the survey (n=150) in Fortaleza, CE 2016.

	Institutionalised		Not institutionalised		Total		P
	N	%	N	%	N	%	
Self-assessment of health							
Very good/Good	50	50%	21	42%	70	46,7%	p=0.22
Regular	31	31%	23	46%	54	36%	
Bad/Very bad	19	19%	7	14%	26	17,3%	
Hospitalisation in the last year							
Yes	14	14%	7	14%	21	14%	p=0.59 fisher
No	86	86%	43	86%	129	86%	
Fall in the last year							
Yes	33	33%	16	32%	49	32,7%	p=0.52
No	67	67%	34	68%	101	67,3%	
Number of illnesses							p=0.017*
chronicles							
none	17	17%	4	8%	21	14%	
1 a 3	77	77%	36	72%	113	75,3%	
more than 4	6	6%	10	20%	16	10,7%	
Polypharmacy							
Yes	63	63%	27	54%	90	60%	p=0.28
No	37	37%	23	46%	60	40%	
Self-medication							
Yes	44	44%	35	70%	79	47,3%	p=0.0026*
No	56	56%	15	30%	71	52,7%	
Use of inappropriate medicines for the elderly							
Yes	19	19%	14	28%	33	22%	p=0.20
No	81	81%	36	72%	117	78%	
Use of teas, herbs							

Yes	52	52%	29	56,9%	81	53,3%	p=0.48
No	48	48%	21	43,1%	69	46,7%	

Source: PINTO; OLIVEIRA NETO; BRAGA, 2017.

Self-medication was found in 47.3 per cent of patients, 70 per cent of whom were assisted at Nami.

Inappropriate medication use was observed in 33 (22%) patients, representing a prevalence of 19% of institutionalised patients and 28% of non-institutionalised patients.

While the use of teas or herbs was observed in 53.3 per cent of the sample, of which 52 per cent represented its use by by institutionalised patients and 56% by non-institutionalised patients.

Among the natural medicines found, the use of tea prevailed with 61.72%, followed by homemade syrup, popularly known as lambedor in the region, with 29.62% and honey with 22.22% of the cases, all of which prevailed in institutionalised patients.

Table 1. Medicines not recommended for the elderly and with options for prescribing other safer drugs according to the Beers - Fick criteria and marketed in Brazil.

Thioridazine	Indomethacin

Barbiturates (except phenobarbital) **Benzodiazepines** Lorazepam > 3.0 mg/day Alprazolam > 2.0 mg/day Chlordiazepoxide Diazepam Clorazepate Flurazepam **Fluoxetine (daily)** Amitriptyline **Antihistamines** Chlorpheniramine	Naproxen Piroxicam **Laxatives** Bisacodyl Sacred cascara Mineral oil **Anorexics** **Amphetamines** Chlorpropamide Non-associated oestrogens (oral) Thyroid extract Methyltestosterone
ifenidramine Hydroxyzine Ciproeptadine Tripelenamine Dexchlorpheniramine Promethazine Amiodarone Digoxin > 0.125 mg/day (except in atrial arrhythmias)	Nitrofurantoin Ferrous sulphate Cimetidine Ketorolac Ergot and ciclandelata **Miorelaxants** **and** **antispasmodics**

Disopyramide	Carisoprodol
Methyldopa	Chlorzoxazone
Clonidine	Cyclobenzaprine
Nifedipine	Orphenadrine
Doxazosin	Oxybutynin
Dipyridamole	Hyoscyamine
Ticlopidine	Propantheline
Non-hormonal anti-inflammatory drugs	Belladonna alkaloids
	Meperidine

Table 3 - Profile of elderly people with polypharmacy (n=91) among institutionalised and non-institutionalised patients in Fortaleza, CE, 2016.

Polypharmacy							
	Institutionalised		**Not institutionalised**		**Total**		**p-value**
	N	%	**N**	%	**N**	**%**	
Sex							
Female	26	40,63%	21	77,78%	47	51,64%	p=0.0012
Male	38	59,38%	6	22,22%	44	48,36%	
Age group							
60 a 74	38	59,38%	18	66,67%	56	61.54%	p=0.51
75 or more	26	40,63%	9	33,33%	35	38,46%	
Education							
Did not study	19	29,69%	2	7,41%	21	23,07%	
up to 4 years	19	29,69%	16	59,26%	35	38,46%	p=0.03
5 to 8 years	12	18,75%	5	18,52%	17		

more than 8 years	14 21,88%	4 14,81%	18,68% 18 19,78%	
Marital status				
No mate	60 93,75%	9 33,33%	69 75,82%	p<0.0001
With a mate	4 6,25%	18 66,67%	22 24,17%	
Income				
Up to 1 salary	51 83,61%	9 37,50%	60 65,93%	P<0.0001
> of 1 salary	10 16,37%	15 52,50%	25 27,47%	
NS/NR	3	3	3 0,03%	
Working conditions				p=0.022 Fisher
Inactive	61 95,31%	19 70,37%	80 87,91%	
Active	3 4,69%	8 29,63%	11 12,08%	
Hospitalisation in the last year				p=0.57 Fisher
Yes	9 14,06%	4 14,81%	13 14,28%	
No	55 85,94%	23 85,19%	78 85,71%	
Fall in the last year				
Yes	18 28,13%	15 55,56%	33 36,26%	p=0.012
No	46 71,88%	12 44,44%	58 63,73%	
Number of chronic diseases				p=0.10
none	10 15,63%	1 0,03%	11 12,08%	
1 a 3	50 78,13%	20 74,07%	70 76,92%	
4 or more	4 6,25%	6 22,22%	10 10,98%	
Self-medication				
Yes	25 39,06%	25 92,59%	50 54,94%	p<0.0001
No	39 60,94%	2 7,41%	41 45,05%	
Use of inappropriate				p=0.8

medication for the elderly				
Yes	15 23,44%	7 25,93%	22 24,17%	
No	49 76,56%	20 74,07%	69 75,82%	
Use of teas or herbs				
Yes	34 53,13%	19 70,37%	53 58,24%	p=0.12
No	30 46,88%	8 29,63%	38 41,75%	
Total	64 70,32%	27 29,67%	91	

Source: PINTO; OLIVEIRA NETO; BRAGA, 2017.

Table 3 shows the profile of patients with polypharmacy among institutionalised and non-institutionalised patients. In the group of institutionalised patients with polypharmacy, males predominated, totalling 38 patients (59.38%).

In the non-institutionalised group, 21 patients (77.78%) were female. In both groups, there was a higher prevalence of polypharmacy among patients with less schooling: 56 (61.53%) had not studied or had up to 4 years of schooling.

Only 14 elderly people (15.38%) with polypharmacy had their self-rated health classified as poor or very poor. Regarding inappropriate medication for the elderly, rates of 23.44% and 25.93% were found respectively in institutionalised and non-institutionalised patients with polypharmacy.

In the logistic regression analysis, age was a risk factor for polypharmacy (p=0.007, with Exp (B) 1.07 CI 1.019-1.12) and the number of chronic diseases (p=0.013, with Exp (B) 1.45 CI 1.083-1.942).

Table 4 - Frequency of the 21 medicines most used by the sample studied.

Medicines	N°	%	**Classification ATC (5th Level)**
Losartan	70	7,09%	C09CA01
Simvastatin	56	5,50%	C10AA01
Omeprazole	50	4,80%	A02BC01
Acetyl salicylic acid	49	4,72%	B01AC06
Metformin	31	2,75%	A10BA02
Anlodipine	25	2,12%	C08CA01
Hydrochlorothiazide	22	1,81%	C03AA03
Carbonate of calcium and Vitamin D	19	1,51%	A11AA02
Citalopram	17	1,31%	N06AB04
Atenolol	15	1,12%	C07AB03
Enalapril	14	1,02%	C09AA02
Gliclazide	13	0,93%	A10BB09
Carvedilol	12	0,83%	C07AG02
Furosemide	12	0,83%	C03CA01

Lactulose	12	083%	A06AD11
Alendronate	11	074%	M05BA04
Thiamine	11	0,74%	A11DA01
Levothyroxine	10	0,65%	H03AA01
Risperidone	10	0,65%	N05AX08
Captopril	9	0,56%	C09AA01
Cilostazol	9	0,56%	C04AX33
Total	477	61,00 %	

Source: PINTO; OLIVEIRA NETO; BRAGA, 2017.

Table 4 shows that of the 21 medicines most used by the elderly in the study, 11 (55%) were for the Cardiovascular and Blood Systems (Group C and Group B - AAS), with Losartan being the most used medicine and being used by 70 patients (46.6%), followed by Simvastatin being used by 56 patients (37.3%). The second most frequent class was Food Tract and Metabolism drugs (Group A), with Omeprazole as the main representative in use by 50 interviewees (33.3%).

Table 5 - The 11 unsuitable medicines for the elderly according to the Beers - Fick criteria found in the sample.

Unsuitable medicines for the elderly	**N**	%
Alprazolam	8	22,85%
Diazepam	4	11,42%
Amitriptyline	4	11,42%
Fluoxetine	4	11,42%

Ferrous sulphate	4	11,42%
Digoxin	3	8,57%
Doxazosin	3	8,57%
Oxybutynin	2	5,71%
Amiodarone	1	2,85%
Clonidine	1	2,85%
Cyclobenzaprine	1	2,85%
Total:	35	100%

Source: PINTO; OLIVEIRA NETO; BRAGA, 2017.

22% (33) of the sample used at least one medication that was unsuitable for the elderly and 2 patients (1.33%) used two of these drugs. A total of 11 different drugs were observed, totalling 35 prescriptions.

Benzodiazepines had the highest proportion of use (34.27%), followed by tricyclics, selective serotonin reuptake inhibitors and anti-anaemic drugs, each with 11.42% of the sample using them (Table 5).

Table 6. Possible consequences of potentially inappropriate medication for the elderly found in the sample.

Alprazolam Diazepam	Sedation; possibility of falls and fractures
Amitriptyline	Anticholinergic effects and orthostatic

	hypotension
Fluoxetine	CNS stimulation, agitation and sleep disturbances
Ferrous sulphate	Significant increase in the incidence of constipation
Digoxin	Increased risk of digitalis toxicity
Doxazosin	Hypotension, tachycardia and palpitation
Oxybutynin	Anticholinergic effects; questionable effectiveness at doses tolerated by the elderly
Cyclobenzaprine	Anticholinergic effects; questionable effectiveness at doses tolerated by the elderly
Clonidine	High risk of orthostatic hypotension, depression and sedation
Amiodarone	QT interval changes; severe arrhythmias, such as torsades de pointes

Source: BEERS-FICK, 2003.

CHAPTER 4

DISCUSSION

When analysing sociodemographic variables, there was a predominance of females (54%) in the total sample (150 patients), although there was a discrepancy between the preponderance of the sexes in the two institutions. In the outpatient setting, 76% were women, and among the institutionalised patients, 57% were men.

The prevalence of females at the outpatient clinic may be related to the fact that they have a worse self-reported functional state of health, a greater number of depressive symptoms and hospitalisations, as well as being more concerned about their health and seeking services more than men, making them more likely to actively seek medical attention and medication.

The prevalence of males among the institutionalised elderly in the sample differs from other similar studies, and is explained by the number of women excluded from the study because they were unable to answer the questionnaire or were unaware of their medication.

The prevalence of the 60-74 age group, regardless of gender, is similar to the results obtained in studies carried out in Minas Gerais and São Paulo on patients using the public health system (LOYOLA et al., 2006; OLIVEIRA et al., 2009), but differs from what has been found in other studies and in population projections that point to the high growth of the very elderly population, over 80 years of age (CAMARANO et al., 2010).

The majority of the elderly in the study used polypharmacy in both institutions: 63% among the institutionalised and 54% among the non-institutionalised. The higher prevalence of polypharmacy in LTM is justified by the greater number of elderly people over 75, which predisposes them to greater susceptibility to comorbidities, greater severity of illnesses and a decline in functional status.

In this context, it is generally necessary to prescribe a greater amount of medication for clinical stabilisation.

The factors that showed a statistically significant relationship ($p < 0.05$) with polypharmacy were being female, not having a partner, receiving a lower monthly income (up to 1 minimum wage), having less schooling (up to 4 years), not working and self-medicating.

When analysing the practice of self-medication, 47.33% of the sample self-medicated, with a higher prevalence in outpatient settings (70%) than in long-term care facilities (44%). Patients treated at the Nami were even more likely to use medications that were unsuitable for the elderly.

These results can be explained by the greater control of medication in the LTM due to the monitoring by a multi-professional health team, such as geriatricians and psychiatrists, pharmacists and nursing staff. It should also be borne in mind that outpatients have easier access to medications that can be purchased without a prescription.

Among the medicines unsuitable for the elderly, the main classes found in the results were: Benzodiazepines (Alprazolam and Diazepam), Antidepressants (Amitriptyline and Fluoxetine) and Ferrous Sulphate.

These results differ from those found in the SABE (Health, Well-being and Ageing) study, a population-based cross-sectional study carried out in 2006 which assessed 1258 elderly people in the city of São Paulo. In this study, it was observed that the inappropriate medicines used by the population were predominantly classified as drugs related to the cardiovascular system, followed by those related to the central nervous system (CASSONI, 2011).

In general, the classes of drugs most often found to be unsuitable for the elderly in similar studies are those for the cardiovascular system and the central nervous system (HUFFENBAECHER, et al., 2012; STROHER, et al., 2014).

The preponderance of drugs related to the central nervous system over those related to the cardiovascular system in this study may be related to the higher prevalence of institutionalised elderly people in the sample, because in these patients, the distance from the family environment, the loss of a spouse and the greater number of comorbidities corroborate the development of psychiatric disorders, such as major depression and generalised anxiety disorder.

With regard to the quantity of medication, the interviewees used, on average, less than the average (7.2 to 8.1) per patient in the United States and more than the average (4.7 and 4.6) of other studies in Brazil (DANILOW et al., 2007; BRODERICK et al., 1997).

With regard to the medicines prescribed and according to the ATC classification, the majority of the elderly used medicines that act on the cardiovascular system, followed by those that act on the digestive system and metabolism, and this result is similar to that found in other Brazilian studies on medicalisation in elderly patients (ACURCIO et al., 2009; MARIN et al., 2008; ROZENFELD et al., 2003; COELHO FILHO et al., 2004; LUCCHETI et al., 2010).

As for the use of teas, herbs and homeopathic medicines, 53.33 per cent of the sample used homemade teas and syrups, regionally known as "lickers".

The percentage of use of these substances was similar between the two populations studied. The use of homeopathic substances was not observed in any of the populations studied.

In a study carried out among community-dwelling elderly people in the Federal District, 70 per cent of the sample used teas, home remedies and herbal medicines

(TARQUINIO et al., 2011).

In a household survey of elderly people carried out in Fortaleza, the use of home medication (8.1 per cent) was lower than that found in this study (COELHO FILHO, 2004).

The use of these substances should be known to the doctor, as they can cause interactions, especially with antihypertensive, hypoglycaemic and anticoagulant drugs, as well as other medicines that are used continuously (ALEXANDRE et al., 2008).

Another cross-sectional study found a prevalence of polypharmacy of 30.8 per cent among elderly people in a long-stay institution in São Paulo (GAUTÉRIO et al., 2012).

In Goiânia, a population-based study found that the prevalence of polypharmacy was 26.4 per cent, self-medication 35.7 per cent and 24.6 per cent of the elderly consumed medication considered inappropriate for their age group, according to the Beers-Fick criteria, with greater self-medication being related to lower levels of schooling and poorer self-perception of health (SANTOS et al., 2013). In general, where there is polypharmacy, there is self-medication and the use of inappropriate medicines.

In São Paulo, the prevalence of polypharmacy with associated factors in the elderly was 36 per cent.

The variables most associated with polypharmacy were female gender, age 75 or over, higher income, being in work, regular or poor self-rated health, presence of hypertension, diabetes, rheumatic disease and heart problems. In addition, it was found that using only the public health system was associated inversely with polypharmacy (CARVALHO et al., 2012).

In Quixadá, Ceará, a cross-sectional study of elderly people living in urban areas found a prevalence of 70.6% of polypharmacy among the elderly, more prevalent among females (66.4%), elderly people with a family income of more than one minimum wage, two or more self-reported chronic conditions and regular or poor self-perceived quality of life (SILVA et al., 2012).

CHAPTER 5

CONCLUSION

This study characterised elderly residents of a long-term care institution and elderly people from the community undergoing outpatient medical care in terms of their use of medication, and found polypharmacy in 60% of the total sample, with a higher prevalence among institutionalised elderly people than among non-institutionalised people (63% versus 54%).

Among the variables with which a statistically significant relationship was observed with polypharmacy were female gender, not having a partner, receiving a lower monthly income, having less schooling, not working and self-medication.

The drugs most used by the participants were from the Cardiovascular and Blood Systems class (Group C and Group B - AAS), followed by Food Tract and Metabolism drugs (Group A).

The use of inappropriate medication for the elderly was found in 22% of the population, with a predominance of this practice in the non-institutionalised elderly (28%)

over the institutionalised (19%), with the majority of the classes of these drugs being related to the central nervous system.

The vulnerability of the elderly to adverse events related to the use of medicines is high, due to the complexity of clinical problems, the need for multiple agents and the pharmacokinetic and pharmacodynamic changes inherent in ageing.

This study contributes to an understanding of the reality of the elderly, especially the institutionalised, in relation to the use of medicines, providing a basis for health professionals to encourage the rational use of medicines.

CHAPTER 6

REFERENCES

ALEXANDRE, R.F; BAGATINI, F.; SIMÕES, C. M. O. Interactions between drugs and herbal medicines based on ginkgo or ginseng. Revista brasileira de farmacognosia. v.18(1) João Pessoa Jan./Mar. 2008.

ALMEIDA, O. P. et al. Predictors and clinical consequences of the use of multiple medications among elderly people treated at an outpatient mental health service. Revista Brasileira de Psiquiatria, v. 21, p. 152-157, 1999.

BEERS, M. H. et al. Explicit criteria for determining inappropriate medication use in nursing home residents. UCLA Division of Geriatric Medicine. Arch Intern Med, v. 151, n. 9, p. 1825-32, Sep 1991.

BEERS, M. H. Explicit criteria for determining potentially inappropriate medication use by the elderly.

An update. Arch Intern Med, v. 157, n. 14, p. 1531-6, Jul 28 1997.

BRODERICK E. Prescribing patterns for nursing home residents in the US. The reality and the vision. Drugs Aging 1997; 11(4):255-60

CAMARANO AA, Mello e Leitão J. Introduction. In: Camarano AA, editor. Long-term care for the elderly: a new social risk to be assumed? Rio de Janeiro: IPEA; 2010. p. 13-37.

CARVALHO, M. F. C. et al. Polypharmacy among the elderly in the city of São Paulo - SABE Study. Revista Brasileira de Epidemiologia, v. 15, p. 817827, 2012.

CASSONI, T. C. J. Use of potentially inappropriate medication by elderly people in the municipality of São Paulo - SABE Study - Health, Well-being and Ageing (Master's thesis). São Paulo: School of Public Health,

University of São Paulo; 2011.

COELHO FILHO, João Macêdo; MARCOPITO, Luiz Francisco; CASTELO, Adauto. Profile of medication use by the elderly in an urban area in the north-east of Brazil. Rev. Saúde Pública, São Paulo, v. 38,n. 4,p. 557-564, Aug. 2004.

DAL PIZZOL, T. D. S. et al. Medication use among elderly people living in urban and rural areas of a municipality in southern Brazil: a population-based study. Cadernos de Saúde Pública, v. 28, p. 104-114, 2012.

DANILOW MZ, Moreira ACS. Epidemiological, sociodemographic and psychosocial profile of institutionalised elderly people in the Federal District. Communication in health sciences 2007; 18(1):9- 16.

DIEDERICHS, C.; BERGER, K.; BARTELS, D. B. The measurement of multiple chronic diseases--a systematic review on existing multimorbidity indices. J Gerontol A Biol Sci Med Sci, v. 66, n. 3, p. 301-11, Mar 2011.

FICK, D. M. et al. Updating the Beers criteria for potentially inappropriate medication use in older adults: results of a US consensus panel of experts. Arch Intern Med, v. 163, n. 22, p. 2716-24, Dec 8-22 2003.

FLORES, L. M.; MENGUE, S. S. Use of medicines by the elderly in a region of southern Brazil. Revista de Saúde Pública, v. 39, p. 924-929, 2005.

GAUTÉRIO, D. P. et al. Characterisation of elderly medication users living in a long-term care institution. Revista da Escola de Enfermagem da USP, v. 46, p. 1394-1399, 2012.

GOMES HO, Caldas CP. Inappropriate use of medication by the elderly: polypharmacy and its effects.

Revista Hospital Universitário Pedro Ernesto. 2008; (1): 88-99

GORZONI, Milton Luiz; FABBRI, Renato Moraes Alves; PIRES, Sueli Luciano. Potentially inappropriate medicines for the elderly. Rev. Assoc. Med. Bras., São Paulo, v. 58, n. 4, p. 442446, Aug. 2012.

HOLT S, Schmiedl S, Thurmann PA. Potentially inappropriate medications in the elderly: the PRISCUS List. Dtsch Arztebl Int. 2010;107(31- 32):543-51.

HUFFENBAECHER, P.; VARALLO, F. R.; MASTROIANNI, P. C. Inadequate medication for the elderly in the family health strategy. Rev. Ciênc. Ext. v.8, n.3, p.56-67, 2012.

LUCCHETTI, G. et al. Factors associated with the use of psychotropic drugs in elderly nursing homes. Revista de Psiquiatria do Rio Grande do Sul, v. 32, p. 38-

43, 2010.

MARIN, M. J. S. et al. Nursing diagnoses of elderly people who use multiple medications. Revista da Escola de Enfermagem da USP, v. 44, p. 47-52, 2010.

MEDEIROS-SOUZA, P. et al. Diagnosis and control of polypharmacy in the elderly. Revista de Saúde Pública, v. 41, p. 1049-1053, 2007.

OLIVEIRA, C. A. P. D. et al. Characterisation of medicines prescribed to the elderly in the Family Health Strategy. Cadernos de Saúde Pública, v. 25, p. 1007-1016, 2009.

WORLD HEALTH ORGANISATION (OMS). ICD-10 - International Statistical Classification of Diseases and Related Health Problems. 10ª revision. Brasília: WHO Collaborating Centre for the Classification of Diseases in Portuguese; 1995.

PASSARELLI, M. C.; JACOB-FILHO, W.; FIGUERAS, A. Adverse drug reactions in an elderly hospitalised population: inappropriate prescription is a leading cause. Drugs Aging, v. 22, n. 9, p. 767-77, 2005.

PENTEADO, P. T. P. et al. The use of medication by the elderly. Visão Acadêmica, Curitiba, v.3, n.1, p.35-42, Jan./June2002.

ROZENFELD S., Fonseca MJM, Acurcio FA. Drug utilisation and polypharmacy among the elderly: a survey in Rio de Janeiro City, Brazil. Pan Am J Public Health 2008; 23:34-43.

SANTOS, T. R. A. et al. Consumption of medicines by the elderly, Goiânia, Brazil. Revista de Saúde Pública, v. 47, p. 94-103, 2013.

SILVA, G. D. O. B. et al. Use of continuous

medication and associated factors in the elderly of Quixadá, Ceará. Revista Brasileira de Epidemiologia, v. 15, p. 386-395, 2012.

SILVIA REGINA, S. Polypharmacy: interactions and adverse reactions in the use of medicines by the elderly. Revista Brasileira de Enfermagem, v. 63, n. 1, 2010.

STROHER, Amanda; ZUBIOLI, Arnaldo. Prevalence of potentially inappropriate medicines for the elderly among those standardised at the Maringá regional university hospital according the Beers-Fick criteria. Infarma - Ciências Farmacêuticas, [S.l.], v. 26, n. 1, p. 4-10, mar. 2014.

TARQUINIO, R. A. et al. Home pharmaceutical care in a group of elderly people in the Federal District. Cenarium Pharmacêutico, Year 4, No. 4, May/Nov 2011.

TAYLOR, A. W. et al. Multimorbidity - not just an

older person's issue. Results from an Australian biomedical study. BMC Public Health, v. 10, p. 718, 2010.

WORLD HEALTH ORGANISATION (WHO). The safety of medicines in public health programmes: pharmacovigilance an essential tool. Geneva; 2006.

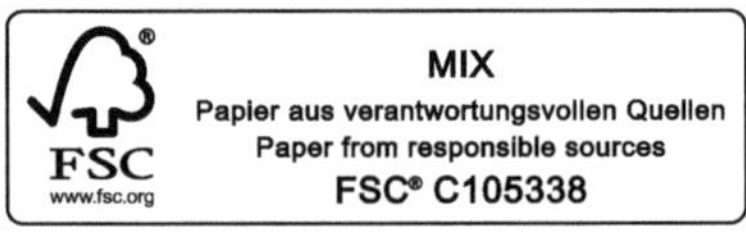

Printed by Books on Demand GmbH, Norderstedt / Germany